DR. POOP'S 30 DAY GUT RESET

YOU WILL ROCK YOUR BOWELS! 5,000 YEARS
OF AYURVEDIC MEDICINAL WISDOM ON
HOW TO POOP BETTER AND STOP GETTING
CONSTIPATED.

DR. POOP

YOU WILL ROCK BOOKS

CONTENTS

DISCLAIMER

Disclaimer Notice:

The information presented in this book is intended solely for educational and entertainment purposes. It is not intended to diagnose, treat, cure, or prevent any disease or health condition. The content is based on a combination of traditional Ayurvedic practices, herbal remedies, personal experiences, and publicly available research. While every effort has been made to ensure accuracy, the information may not reflect the most current developments in medical science or integrative health.

The practices and suggestions outlined in this book are not a substitute for professional medical advice, diagnosis, or treatment. Always seek the advice of your physician or another qualified health provider with any questions you may have regarding a medical condition or before beginning any new health routine, dietary change, or supplement regimen. Never disregard professional medical advice or delay in seeking it because of something you have read in this book.

The author and publisher are not licensed medical professionals, dietitians, or healthcare practitioners. The character "Dr.

Poop" is a fictional persona created for humor and educational storytelling. He is not a licensed doctor. The use of this character is not intended to mislead or imply professional credentials.

By reading this book, you acknowledge that the author and publisher are not liable for any adverse effects, loss, injury, or damage allegedly arising directly or indirectly from the application or interpretation of the content within. Use of any information provided is at your own risk.

For personalized medical advice, please consult with a licensed healthcare provider. Ayurveda is a complementary system of health that may not be appropriate for everyone and is not recognized as a substitute for Western medical treatment.

To my sisters who have struggled with constipation.
I hope this book provides you both relief.

And to Ayurveda, meaning "knowledge of life" in Sanskrit, a holistic
healing system developed in India over 5,000 years ago.

INTRODUCTION

L et's start with something radical.

You are not broken. You don't need a lifetime supply of fiber powders, a pyramid of probiotic pills, or another fear-based cleanse. You're not lazy, weak, or doomed to live with bloating and constipation. You're just out of rhythm with your body. We've all been there.

In my house, we believe regular pooping is not a luxury, it's a right. A glorious, grounding, serotonin boosting right. And yes, you can reclaim it. Somewhere along the way, we stopped listening to our bodies.

We started eating in cars, scrolling on toilets, sprinting through life powered by caffeine, cortisol, and convenience. We normalized skipping breakfast and stress-snacking by 3 p.m., crashing into bed without ever once asking our gut: How are you doing?

What was once a predictable part of daily life became unpredictable, embarrassing, or just plain absent. The signals got scrambled. The rituals got forgotten. And the conversations about gut health were replaced with TikToks pushing detox teas and tummy gummies.

No wonder your digestive system is confused. But here's the good news, your gut wants to get back in sync.

You just have to *show it* how, and that's what I'm here for.

Why This Book Exists

Let's be honest: most of us have Googled "how to poop faster" in a moment of desperation, or stared into the distance on the toilet wondering, "why is nothing happening?". Maybe you've avoided jeans for days because of bloating, or felt a familiar pressure build at the worst possible time, like in the middle of a work meeting or a long car ride.

You are not alone.

This book is your antidote to that frustration. Not with fear, shame, or quick fixes, but with rituals that actually work.

It's a 30-day plan to teach your body how to move again, naturally and consistently.

What This Book Isn't

Let's set the ground rules:

- This is not a shame spiral. Your experience is valid. Your discomfort is real. Your struggle is not your fault.
- This is not a crash cleanse. No starvation. No juice-only weeks. No disappearing into the bathroom every 30 minutes.
- This is not pseudoscience. Every ritual is either time-tested through ancient wisdom or backed by modern studies. Often, both.

What you'll find here is a balanced, joyful, and practical plan. You'll laugh, you'll learn, and by the end, you'll poop better. Every. Single. Day.

Who This Book Is For

You don't need a doctor's note or a diagnosis to deserve relief. This is for the people who:

- Haven't had a satisfying poop in days (or weeks)
- Feel bloated after every meal
- Panic when a bathroom isn't nearby
- Have been pregnant, are postpartum, or are navigating hormonal shifts
- Tried every social media gut hack with zero results
- Work long hours, sit all day, or rarely feel "the urge"

Whether you're a new parent, an overworked entrepreneur, an athlete, a teacher, an uber driver, or someone who just wants to enjoy a meal without regretting it, this reset is for you.

Why It Works: The Three Pillars

This reset combines three powerful systems to guide your transformation:

1. AYURVEDA

With over 5,000 years of wisdom, Ayurveda teaches that digestion (Agni) is the root of health. When it burns bright, we feel energized, clear, and regular. When it's weak, we feel heavy, foggy, and stuck. Through spices, oils, breathing, and timing, you'll restore your digestive rhythm.

Pronounced *eye-your-VAY-duh*, it is one of the oldest healing systems on Earth. Originating in India, this ancient science is all about balance. It teaches that true health isn't just about what you eat, but when you eat, how you feel while eating, and how well your body actually digests it.

At the center of Ayurveda is a fiery concept called **Agni**, which literally means "digestive fire." Imagine your gut as a little furnace: when it's burning strong, you feel clear, energized, and regular. When the fire gets weak, digestion slows, toxins build up, and you feel bloated, foggy, and constipated. (Sound familiar?)

Ayurveda's mission is to keep that fire hot, happy, and in tune: not too much, not too little.

The Three Doshas (A.K.A. Your Body's Operating System)

According to Ayurveda, every person is made up of three vital energies, or **Doshas**, called **Vata**, **Pitta**, and **Kapha**. Each dosha has its own personality, tendencies, and poop problems:

• **Vata** is air and space. Think light, dry, and cold. Vata folks may have constipation, anxiety, and gas that could clear a room. They do best with warmth, grounding routines, and cooked foods.

• **Pitta** is fire and water. These folks are hot, intense, and driven, but can be prone to loose stools, acid reflux, and irritation. They benefit from cooling herbs and calming rituals.

• **Kapha** is earth and water. Think heavy, stable, and slow. Kapha digestion can be sluggish, leading to bloat, weight gain, and that post-meal "I-need-a-nap" feeling. Spices, movement, and warmth are their best friends.

You're probably a mix of all three, but one or two usually dominate. Don't stress about memorizing them. Ayurveda is a way of life, and this book spotlights each section with its Ayurvedic principle.

2. HERBAL & NATURAL REMEDIES

We tap into gentle, time-tested remedies like warm lemon water, ginger, olive oil, belly massage, and castor oil packs. These tools support the body, without causing dependence or discomfort.

When your gut's off, the whole body knows it. Your brain, your skin, your mood, and even your sleep are affected. That's where nature steps in. Herbal and natural remedies are powerful tools that have been used for centuries (long before laxatives came in bright pink bottles). They don't just force your body into action—they support your body's *own* rhythm so it can do what it was made to do: digest, detox, and poop with ease.

Herbal remedies are the plant-powered MVPs of your gut-healing journey. They work gently but deeply, helping to calm inflammation, boost bile flow, stimulate digestion, and relax tension in your belly and bowels. You're not just masking symptoms—you're nourishing your system from the inside out.

Some herbs are true classics. **Ginger** and **fennel** warm the digestive tract and ease bloating. **Triphala**, a staple in Ayurvedic medicine, is famous for helping you go without the "uh-oh" urgency.

There are also **minerals** like **magnesium citrate**, which acts like a gentle flush for the colon without harsh side effects. And let's not forget the role of **oils**, like castor oil, used in traditional massage to stimulate the gut and move toxins out of the system.

The best part is you'll find many of these remedies in your spice cabinet, tea drawer, or local grocery aisle. This book will show you how to use them in simple, doable ways, like sippable teas and bedtime habits that help your body heal while you rest.

A few notes before we dive in:

• Herbs take time. Don't expect a magic poop 5 minutes after sipping a tea. Think of it as planting seeds for long-term balance.

• Less is often more. Start small, be consistent, and pay attention to how your body feels.

• And always—yes, always—drink water when adding fiber or herbs. Hydration is half the battle.

This book weaves in herbal and natural remedies in simple, non-intimidating ways.

3. MODERN GUT SCIENCE

When it comes to your gut, science has finally caught up to what ancient medicine has known all along: your poop isn't just about food, it's about your entire ecosystem.

Modern gut science has exploded in the last decade, giving us incredible tools to understand how digestion affects everything from your brain to your immune system. At the center of this research is something called the **microbiome**: a massive colony of bacteria (both good and bad) that live in your gut and play a starring role in how your body functions. They help digest food, regulate mood, balance hormones, and even control inflammation.

Another key player is the The **gut-brain axis**. This is the direct communication line between your stomach and your central nervous system. That anxious, twisty belly feeling before a big meeting? That's not just nerves. It's your gut and brain chatting, and often, your gut is doing the shouting.

Science also now confirms that seemingly random things like your **posture, sleep patterns, hydration**, and even the **time of day** you eat can deeply affect digestion. Slouching slows gut motility. Late-night snacking messes with your circadian rhythm. Stress triggers gut spasms. Dehydration? That's constipation's best friend.

This book blends modern science and ancient wisdom in a way that's actually doable. We're not here to overwhelm you with peer-reviewed jargon. We're here to help you build habits that *work*, whether they come from 5,000 year old medicine, a tea leaf, or your grandma's kitchen.

Here's what you can expect from the science-backed side of this guide:

• Movement that stimulates digestion (without needing a gym)

• Foods that repair your gut lining and feed good bacteria

• Posture and breathwork techniques that calm your belly and your brain

This isn't about choosing one system over another. It's about layering the best of both worlds, Eastern and Western, old and new, into a gut-loving reset that feels natural, works quickly, and sticks with you long after Day 30.

What to Expect Each Week

The 30-day plan is broken into four clear, compound-building phases:

Week 1: Flush the Funk

Hydrate.

Cleanse.

Awaken your digestive fire.

Week 2: Feed the Gut Garden

Nourish your microbiome.

Add diversity, fiber, and pre/probiotics.

Week 3: Poop Like a Pro

Lock in timing, improve posture, and activate your nervous system.

Week 4: Maintain the Movement

Build a sustainable routine for daily gut peace.

Each chapter includes easy-to-follow rituals, quick explanations of why they work, and encouraging tools to help you stay consistent. (Yes, you'll love it.) This creates habit stacking, where small, intentional actions begin to rewire your rhythm and compound.

How to Use This Book

By reading each chapter at the start of the week, you can pick your rituals, practice them daily, reflect, tweak, and feel the shift.

You don't need to do everything. Start with three rituals a day, commit to the process, and give your body the rhythm it craves.

Some rituals may feel weird at first. Others might change your life overnight. You'll start seeing patterns, this tea makes a difference, that posture helps, this food sets things off. Trust the process.

There's no failing. Only learning. I've also added a few bonus chapters too!

What It Is

This isn't a strict program. It's a rhythm. A reset. A gentle invitation to listen to your body in a new way. You don't need to become a digestive overachiever or memorize every single ritual. Instead, think of this book as your gut's new best friend, a playbook full of tools, not rules.

Here's the secret: You don't need to do everything. You just need to begin. That is always the hardest part.

Once you commit, you'll be amazed at how much your body will thank you.

Start with three small rituals a day, whatever feels doable. Maybe that's sipping warm lemon water in the morning, trying a squatting posture when you poop, and skipping your phone during bathroom time. Maybe it's a daily belly massage, a probiotic smoothie, and walking after lunch. Whatever it is, commit to it. Your body thrives on rhythm, and the more consistent you are, the more your gut will respond.

Why This Works

Your gut is a fast learner, but it also responds best to consistency. Think of this like tuning an instrument. It takes a little practice and patience, but once you're in sync, everything plays smoother.

Small daily rituals send signals to your body:

"This is your time to rest."

"This is your cue to digest."

"This is your moment to release."

When repeated with care, these cues create a dependable pattern for elimination, energy, and ease. What once felt mysterious or out of control starts to feel manageable, even empowering.

Some rituals may feel strange at first. That's normal.

You might think, "Do I really need to oil my belly?" or "Is this tea actually doing anything?" But keep going. Your body speaks in whispers before it shouts. If you listen closely, you'll start noticing:

- This smoothie keeps things moving.
- That bedtime tea helps me sleep.
- This squat changed my restroom game forever.

You'll build awareness. Patterns. Confidence. And, eventually, progress you can feel in your jeans, your mood, and your energy.

The Big Secret Nobody Tells You

A good poop can change your mood, your day, and your entire sense of well-being.

Your gut influences:

- Mood & Mental Health: Your gut makes 90% of your serotonin. Poop is peace.
- Immunity: 70% of your immune system lives in the gut.
- Hormones: Estrogen and other hormones are regulated here. Constipation throws everything off.
- Skin Health: Breakouts, eczema, and dull skin often start in the colon.
- Energy & Focus: A backed-up gut = sluggish everything.

So no, we're not being dramatic. We're being honest. Your poop matters, probably more than you've ever been told.

Let's Normalize the Conversation

It's time to drop the stigma.

Doctors barely ask about it. Social media skips to the shiny supplements. No one is teaching us how to build sustainable, non-scary habits.

This book flips the script with compassion, science, and a little humor.

Pooping is not gross. It's healing. It's human. It's your body saying: Thank you for taking care of me.

Ready to Begin?

By the end of this 30-day journey, you'll have more than regular bowel movements. You'll have a toolkit for life. You'll feel lighter, clearer, and more connected to your body.

So unclench. Breathe. Laugh a little.

Final Reminder

There's no such thing as failing here. Only learning.

One bad day? It's just feedback. One great poop? Celebrate it. This isn't about perfection. It's about progress, permission, and partnership, with your gut, your breath, and your body.

You're not here to follow a rigid system. You're here to remember what your gut's been trying to tell you all along:

You don't need to be fixed. You just need a rhythm.

So pick your rituals. Set the tone. And begin.

Let's get your gut back on beat.

You will rock your bowels!

Let's begin.

With deepest respect (and a wink),

   - Dr. Poop A.K.A. "Constipation's Worst Nightmare"

P.S. - For every Dr. Poop book sold we will donate a portion of the profits to charities around the world.

Everyone deserves to live healthy.

Buy a book. Help a life.

What Is The Dr. Poop Challenge?

At the end of each chapter, I'll be introducing "The Dr. Poop Challenge", which are action steps for you to take right away. This is designed to prevent information overload and guide you after consuming all the information. Get your family and friends to join the challenge with you to make it more fun!

Tag us **@Youwillrockbooks** on all socials to get featured in The Dr. Poop Challenge!

The Dr. Poop Challenge

Track your rituals in a notebook or notes app. Nothing fancy, just jot down what you tried, what helped, what didn't. Over time, you'll build your own personal poop playbook. It's one of the fastest ways to figure out what works for you.

You can also download your very own free Dr. Poop's 30 Day Gut Reset Tracker with the QR code below.

Now, let's get started with Week 1: Flush the Funk, where we wake up your digestion, clear out the clutter, and ignite your bathroom confidence one glorious poop at a time.

1

WEEK 1: FLUSH THE FUNK

This is your 7-day gut reset to activate natural rhythm, clear out funk, and rehydrate your system from the inside out. Think of it like spring cleaning for your colon, without the crash diets or scary laxatives. You're not flushing everything out. You're inviting everything in: hydration, flow, and regularity.

This Week's Goal

This week, we're hitting the reset button on your digestive system, think of it as a deep clean for your gut without any extreme measures. It's about clearing out the build up, rehydrating, and giving your body the space to reset.

Why It Works

When the gut is stagnant, so is everything else, mood, energy, even immunity. By gently stimulating digestion with warm fluids, gentle detoxifiers, and natural movement, you're reigniting the body's rhythm without triggering stress or strain. This week's practices are designed to lubricate your pipes, reset your nervous system, and restore elimination without forcing it.

Ayurvedic Spotlight

In Ayurveda, elimination is one of the three pillars of health (Traya Upastambha). When you're not pooping regularly, Ama (toxins) build up and clog your system.

This week's focus mirrors the Ayurvedic concept of:

- Supporting Apana Vayu (the downward flow of energy)
- Stimulating Agni (digestive fire)
- Releasing stuck Vata that contributes to dryness, gas, and irregularity

Dr. Poop's Pro Tip

Start this week by taking inventory of your current habits. Are you rushing in the morning? Eating standing up? Skipping hydration? The smallest tweaks this week can have major impact. You don't need to be perfect, just consistent.

THE LEMON FLUSH

What It Is

A warm morning drink made with:

- 1 cup warm water
- ½ fresh lemon (squeezed)
- A pinch of sea salt

Sip it first thing on an empty stomach.

Why It Works

This trio activates your gut's natural rhythm. Warm water hydrates and gently dilates the gut lining, lemon triggers your liver and gallbladder to release bile, and sea salt replenishes electrolytes and minerals. Together, they stimulate peristalsis (the movement that pushes poop through). It's hydration meets activation.

Ayurvedic Spotlight

In Ayurveda, mornings are sacred and the digestive system is most ready to receive. This warm lemon ritual is used to:

- Stimulate Agni (digestive fire)
- Soften and moisten dry stool
- Flush Ama (toxins) accumulated overnight
- Prepare the body for elimination

Sea salt provides grounding earth and water elements, balancing excess Vata. This is a gentle dinacharya (daily practice) to wake up your gut with care.

Dr. Poop's Pro Tip

Add a dash of cayenne or apple cider vinegar if you want to crank up the fire. Or try it with warm coconut water if you're feeling dry or depleted.

THE TRIPHALA OR MAGNESIUM SHOWDOWN

What It Is

Your nighttime gut tune-up. Choose one:

- **Option A:** 1 tsp Triphala powder mixed into warm water, taken 30–60 minutes before bed.
- **Option B:** 200 mg magnesium citrate capsule, also taken before sleep.

Why It Works
Your body detoxifies and repairs itself while you sleep, so giving it gentle support can make a big difference by morning.

- Triphala works by toning the colon and supporting liver detox without creating dependency.
- Magnesium citrate pulls water into the colon, softening stool and stimulating a gentle release, without the urgency of harsher laxatives.

Ayurvedic Spotlight
What is triphala? Triphala is Ayurveda's OG detox blend, made from three fruits that work in harmony:

- **Amla** (Indian Gooseberry): High in Vitamin C, supports immunity and skin health
- **Bibhitaki**: Clears mucus and supports respiratory + gut health
- **Haritaki**: Known as the "king of medicine," improves digestion and longevity

Together, these fruits:

- Balance all three doshas
- Improve gut motility
- Detox the liver and colon
- Promote regular, easy poops without dependency

Triphala is not a cleanse. It's a nightly ritual that honors your body's natural rhythm and clears out the funk without disruption.

Dr. Poop's Pro Tip

If you're sensitive to powders or the taste of herbs, start with magnesium first. Then work your way into Triphala once you've reset your routine.

THE 10-MINUTE POST-MEAL WALK

What It Is

This is a light 10–15 minute walk after eating. You're not power-walking. You're stroll-pooping.

It can be around your block, your kitchen island, or even just standing stretches with slow steps.

Why It Works

Eating stimulates your gastrocolic reflex, the body's natural cue to move food along the digestive tract. Gentle movement boosts this signal, helping your gut prep for smooth elimination. Plus, walking improves circulation, lowers blood sugar, and relieves that "ugh-I-ate-too-much" bloat.

. . .

Ayurvedic Spotlight

In Ayurveda, digestion isn't just about food. It's about flow. After eating, gentle movement supports:

- Activation of Apana Vayu (downward energy)
- Boosted peristalsis (the gut's wave-like motion)
- Soothed nervous system—important for safe elimination

This isn't about burning calories. It's about honoring your digestion and giving it a little post meal nudge.

Dr. Poop's Pro Tip

Pair your post-meal walk with a 5-minute gratitude practice. It's a gut + mood combo that's way more powerful than scrolling your phone after dinner.

THE MAGIC BELLY MASSAGE

What It Is

A simple 1–2 minute clockwise belly massage using warm castor oil.

Start on the lower right side of your belly, move up to your ribs, across to the left, then down, following the path of your colon.

Why It Works

This isn't just self-care, it's gut-care.

- The warmth of the oil calms your nervous system and helps your gut relax.
- Gentle massage encourages colon movement and reduces tension or stagnation.
- Castor oil promotes lymphatic drainage, which helps flush toxins from your system.

Ayurvedic Spotlight

Ayurveda calls this practice Abhyanga, a sacred oil massage used daily to support circulation, immunity, and detoxification.

Castor oil in particular is:

- Deeply penetrating, reaching the tissue layers where toxins can hide
- Naturally anti-inflammatory, which soothes digestive discomfort
- Supportive of gut, liver, and lymph flow, helping everything move downstream

The clockwise motion aligns with the natural path of elimination, gently telling your colon: "Hey, it's okay to let go now."

This isn't just a spa moment, it's a communication tool between your brain and gut.

Dr. Poop's Pro Tip

Wrap a hot water bottle in a towel and place it over your belly after your massage for 10–15 minutes. It's like a spa day for your insides.

THE 3-DAY DAIRY DETOX

What It Is

Cut out all dairy for 3 days, milk, cheese, yogurt, cream, and ice cream.

Don't worry, you can bring it back later. This is a reset, not a life sentence.

Why It Works

Even if you're not lactose intolerant, dairy can still be a mucus forming, heavy food that slows down digestion.

Removing it gives your Agni (digestive fire) a chance to strengthen and reset. Many people notice:

- Less bloating
- Fewer sinus issues
- More regular poops

Ayurvedic Spotlight

In Ayurveda, dairy is classified as:

- Heavy – hard to digest
- Cooling – slows metabolic fire
- Sticky – creates ama (toxic buildup) when not properly digested

That's why traditional Ayurvedic use of dairy is fermented (like yogurt) or clarified (like ghee), forms that are easier for the body to handle.

But most store bought dairy is pasteurized, processed, and stripped of enzymes.

A short detox lets your gut breathe.

You're not saying goodbye to cheese. You're just giving it a long weekend.

Dr. Poop's Pro Tip

Use this week to experiment with non-dairy swaps like oat, almond, or coconut milk. Some brands even make probiotic rich versions to help your gut garden grow.

DR. POOP'S WEEK 1 CHALLENGE

What It Is

This is your official mission for Week 1.

Choose 3 out of the 5 rituals below to commit to daily. If you're feeling bold (and backed up), go for all five.

Your Ritual Menu:

- Morning Lemon Flush
- Nightly Triphala or Magnesium
- 10-Minute Post-Meal Walks
- The Magic Belly Massage
- 3-Day Dairy Detox

Why It Works

Each ritual in Week 1 was designed to gently retrain your gut rhythm, no purging, no pushing, just natural activation.

By choosing your top 3 and sticking with them, you'll:

- Build consistency
- Reduce overwhelm
- See measurable wins without overdoing it

Ayurvedic Spotlight

Ayurveda teaches that awareness is the first medicine. Before recommending herbs or protocols, practitioners observe patterns.

This week, your poop becomes your personal health journal.

Keep a daily log (notes-style is totally fine):

- Timing
- Texture
- Effort level Not great vs Great

Look for insights like:

- Which rituals make you feel lighter?
- What foods bring on the bloat?
- Are you pooping at the same time daily?

Dr. Poop's Pro Tip

Tell someone about your win, even if it's just your reflection.

Try: "I pooped today. And I'm proud."

(Affirmations count as fiber for the soul.)

. . .

Final Word

You just finished your first week of poop re-education.

You didn't just clear out clutter, you started rebuilding trust with your gut.

Up next: **Week 2 – Feed the Gut Garden**

Let's plant some microbial magic.

2

WEEK 2: FEED THE GUT GARDEN

Welcome to Week 2 of Dr. Poop's 30-Day Gut Reset. Now that you've cleared some of the gunk from the pipes, it's time to focus on what comes next: planting.

Think of your gut like soil. When it's been overworked, inflamed, or fed junk for years, it gets dry, cracked, or even barren. That's when things like constipation, gas, skin issues, fatigue, or immune slumps creep in. But with the right nourishment, you can bring it back to life.

This chapter is all about feeding the beneficial bacteria (aka: your gut's gardeners). These tiny organisms help you digest food, absorb nutrients, regulate hormones, reduce inflammation, and yes poop better.

The secret? Food. Real food. And herbs that have been doing this work since before kombucha made it to Whole Foods.

This Week's Goal

Nourish your microbiome, build better bugs, and fuel smooth digestion with real food and ancient herbs.

Why It Works

When you give your gut microbes the fuel they need, fiber, prebiotics, probiotics, and warm, digestible meals, they return the favor by:

- Producing short-chain fatty acids that reduce inflammation
- Strengthening your intestinal lining
- Improving regularity
- Boosting immunity and mood
- Helping you poop without drama

It's like hiring a team of janitors, therapists, and nutritionists... but inside your belly.

Ayurvedic Spotlight

In Ayurveda, your digestive fire Agni is the foundation of health. When it's strong, you feel energized, clear, and regular. When it's weak or erratic, toxins (called ama) build up and cause trouble.

This week focuses on building strong, steady Agni by using:

- Warm, cooked meals to soothe Vata
- Fiber-rich whole foods to keep things moving
- Fermented and living foods to boost friendly flora (beneficial bacteria)

- Calming teas and daily rituals to support detoxification

Ayurveda reminds us that healing isn't just about what you remove, it's about what you add in.

Dr. Poop's Pro Tip

If you're bloated, gassy, or irregular, don't panic. Your gut is adjusting to new foods, habits, and rhythms. Give yourself grace. Hydrate. Keep going. This week is the turning point.

Ready to feed your gut garden? Let's plant some seeds.

MORNING RITUAL: THE BELLY BLISS BREW (CCF TEA)

Goal

Soothe inflammation, gently wake up digestion, and keep your gut warm and humming all day.

What It Is

Think of this as your gut's morning hug in a mug. CCF Tea is a classic Ayurvedic tonic made with three humble seeds that pack serious digestive power: cumin, coriander, and fennel.

Recipe:

- 1 tsp cumin seeds
- 1 tsp coriander seeds
- 1 tsp fennel seeds

- 3 cups water

Bring everything to a gentle boil and let it simmer for 10–15 minutes. Strain and sip warm. You can drink it all in the morning or spread it out throughout the day.

Why It Works

- Cumin helps reduce gas and bloating while kickstarting digestion.
- Coriander is cooling and soothing for inflamed bellies.
- Fennel relieves cramping, calms the gut, and encourages regular poops.

Together, this trio is like a spa treatment for your digestive system. It gently revs up your "Agni" (digestive fire) without caffeine, helping your body metabolize food more efficiently and reduce inflammation from the inside out.

Ayurvedic Spotlight

In Ayurveda, this blend is prized for being "tridoshic," meaning it balances all three doshas (Vata, Pitta, and Kapha):

- Cumin stimulates but doesn't overheat, making it perfect for sluggish digestion (Kapha) or gas and bloating (Vata).
- Coriander cools heat in the GI tract, ideal for heartburn, inflammation, or loose stools (Pitta).
- Fennel helps move things along while easing tension, great for all three doshas.

This tea is often part of a daily dinacharya (routine), especially if your digestion tends to be irregular, overactive, or just plain confused.

Dr. Poop's Pro Tip

Sip this tea warm or hot. Avoid drinking it iced or straight from the fridge, cold drinks can weaken your Agni and slow digestion.

THE ALOE VERA ELIXIR

Goal

Soothe inflammation, cool the gut, and promote smooth, natural elimination without harsh laxatives.

What It Is

Think of this as a gentle gut elixir, a shot of calm for your digestive tract.

The Aloe Vera Shot is a small, simple ritual:

1–2 ounces of food grade aloe vera juice, taken on an empty stomach in the morning or just before bed.

You can sip it straight (if you're brave), mix it with a splash of water or coconut water, or chill it with a slice of lemon to make it taste a bit less... plant-y.

Why It Works

Aloe vera contains powerful anti inflammatory compounds and a gel like consistency that coats the digestive tract like a soothing balm.

What it does:

- Helps repair and hydrate the gut lining
- Eases constipation without forcing the issue (unlike harsh laxatives)
- Supports liver detoxification
- Reduces bloating, heartburn, and irritation
- Helps flush out heat when you're feeling puffy or inflamed

It's particularly great if you've had spicy food, alcohol, or feel like your digestion is "hot and angry."

Ayurvedic Spotlight

In Ayurveda, aloe vera is called Kumari, which translates to "young maiden" symbolizing renewal and vitality. It's a powerful tonic for the skin, gut, liver, and reproductive system. Aloe Vera (Kumari) has the following benefits:

- Cools excess Pitta (inflammation, acidity, heat-related symptoms)
- Nourishes and hydrates dry, depleted tissues
- Promotes smooth elimination without depleting your energy
- Supports liver function and menstrual balance in women

Aloe is ideal when your gut is feeling irritable and when you want something gentle but effective.

Dr. Poop's Pro Tip

- Use only food-grade aloe vera juice (read the label carefully).
- Look for products labeled "inner leaf only" and free from aloin, a natural laxative in the outer leaf that can be harsh.
- Start with 1 oz and work your way up. No need to chug it!
- If you're feeling fancy, mix it with cucumber juice or coconut water for a spa-like shot.

THE MICROBIOME FERTILIZER

Goal

Feed your gut's good bugs, support regularity, and crowd out processed junk, one delicious swap at a time.

What It Is

This is a gentle food upgrade, not a detox or a diet. It's one small swap that delivers big digestive results.

The idea: Replace just one processed carb with a fiber rich whole food during lunch or your afternoon snack.

Try these simple swaps:

- White rice → quinoa or beans
- Crackers → apple slices or carrot sticks with hummus
- Pasta → lentil or chickpea noodles
- Bread → sprouted grain or sweet potato rounds

Why It Works

Your gut bugs eat what you eat. And they love fiber.
Fiber has the following benefits:

- Acts like fertilizer for your microbiome, helping good bacteria grow
- Adds bulk to your stool and helps keep things moving
- Slows blood sugar spikes (so you don't crash and crave more junk)
- Helps regulate appetite, energy, and even mood

Adding even 5 more grams of fiber a day can make a difference in bloating, energy, and yes bathroom consistency.

Ayurvedic Spotlight

While Ayurveda doesn't measure grams of fiber, it's all about wholesome, natural foods that support "sama agni" balanced digestion:

- Legumes, lentils, seasonal fruits, and whole grains like barley and millet are praised for their grounding and stabilizing effects
- These foods balance Vata dosha, the airy energy linked to irregularity and bloating
- Proper food combining, like not mixing fruits and dairy also keeps your gut from getting confused (or gassy)

Ayurveda teaches that digestion begins with the quality of your food and fiber-rich options are considered more "sattvic," or life-giving.

. . .

Dr. Poop's Pro Tip

- Don't go from 10g of fiber to 40g overnight. Your gut will protest.
- Start slow, increase gradually, and add extra water to help things move.
- Want a sweet option? Try chia pudding, roasted chickpeas, or a green banana with almond butter.

ANTI FIGHT-OR-FLIGHT BELLY BREATHING

Goal

Calm your nervous system, activate digestion, and send your gut the signal that it's safe to let go.

What It Is

This is not just "take a deep breath." This is a mini nervous system reboot, right before meals.

Deep belly breathing (aka diaphragmatic breathing) involves slowly inhaling into your lower belly rather than your chest, then gently exhaling to create a full body reset. You're shifting out of fight-or-flight (which shuts down digestion) and into rest and digest mode.

How To Do It

1. Sit down comfortably, feet flat on the floor.
2. Place one hand on your chest, one on your belly.

3. Inhale through your nose for 4 seconds, feeling your belly rise (not your chest).
4. Hold for 4 seconds.
5. Exhale slowly through your mouth for 6 seconds.
6. Repeat for 3–5 rounds, or set a timer for 3–5 minutes.

Try this before meals, before bed, or even on the toilet if things aren't... moving.

Why It Works

Digestion isn't just about what you eat. It's about how your body feels when you eat.

Stress sends cortisol soaring, tightening your gut muscles, drying your colon, and putting your whole digestive system on pause.

Breathing Deeply

- Activates the vagus nerve, which controls your gut-brain communication
- Increases blood flow to your digestive organs
- Signals your body to start producing digestive enzymes and acids
- Relaxes your pelvic floor muscles (yes, even those!)
- Creates a rhythm for elimination

Basically, it's the reset button for your gut, and it's totally free.

Ayurvedic Spotlight

In Ayurveda, breath is known as prana, or life force. The way you breathe directly reflects the way you live.

Rushed, shallow breathing = scattered mind and poor digestion.

Deep, rhythmic breathing = calm mind and strong Agni (digestive fire).

This practice is part of Dinacharya, the daily lifestyle rituals that help your body align with natural rhythms.

Before meals, conscious breathing prepares your gut to receive and process food with grace, not chaos.

Ayurveda doesn't separate digestion and emotion, both are connected. Breathing is how you bridge the two.

Dr. Poop's Pro Tip
  Use the 4-4-6 method:

- Inhale for 4 seconds
- Hold for 4 seconds
- Exhale for 6 seconds

The longer exhale activates your parasympathetic nervous system.

THE SLIP-N-SLIDE SMOOTHIE:

Goal

Boost fiber, hydrate your colon, and plant gut friendly seeds, literally.

What It Is

This smoothie isn't just tasty, it's tactical. We're blending together some of nature's finest gut loving ingredients:

- 1 small kiwi – skin optional, but edible!
- ½ cup papaya – fresh or frozen chunks
- 1 tablespoon ground flaxseed – optional, but powerful
- 1–2 soft medjool dates – natural sweetness + fiber
- 1 teaspoon ghee – Ayurvedic gold (can sub coconut oil if needed)
- ½ cup warm water or unsweetened almond milk

Blend until smooth. Sip slowly in the morning before breakfast or use as your breakfast. This is your daily gut garden in a glass.

Why It Works

- Papaya contains papain, an enzyme that helps break down proteins and soften stool.
- Kiwi is rich in actinidin, a poop promoting enzyme clinically shown to help with regularity.
- Flax is loaded with soluble fiber and omega-3s that help sweep the intestines and ease inflammation.
- Dates add natural sweetness, potassium, and additional fiber for smooth passage.
- Ghee, a clarified butter used in Ayurveda, nourishes the digestive lining and promotes healthy "Agni."

Ayurvedic Spotlight

- Papaya isn't traditionally Ayurvedic, but its gut-soothing enzymes act similarly to pitta balancing herbs.
- Flax offer moist, unctuous properties that help balance Vata the dry, airy dosha often responsible for constipation.
- Dates are considered grounding and nourishing in Ayurveda, helping support elimination without being too stimulating.
- Ghee is revered as a digestive tonic. It lubricates the colon, supports nutrient absorption, and is one of the safest fats for internal use.

In Ayurveda, when your gut lining is dry and your "Agni" is weak, digestion suffers. This smoothie restores moisture, feeds good bacteria, and brings everything back into rhythm.

Dr. Poop's Pro Tip

Drink warm or room temp not ice cold to protect your Agni.

DR. POOP'S WEEK 2 CHALLENGE

Mission: Pick 3 of the 5 rituals to commit to this week. If you're feeling bold, go for all five. This is *your* gut garden, we're just planting the seeds.

What It Is

This week, you're not just "trying to poop more." You're actively re-coding your gut with better bacteria, smarter digestion, and cleaner signals to the rest of your body. Think of these rituals as your fertilizer.

You'll choose from the following:

- Sip The Belly Bliss Brew in the morning to warm up your digestive fire
- Start your day with the Slip-N-Slide Smoothie
- Replace one carb with a fiber rich whole food
- Take a gentle Aloe Vera Elixir before bed or first thing in the morning
- Do 3–5 minutes of Anti Fight-or-Flight Belly Breathing before meals

Just 3 out of 5 gets you results. All 5? That's gut garden glory.

Why It Works

Your body speaks in sensations bloat, fatigue, cravings, mood dips, random skin flares. That's its way of saying, "Hey, something's off."

But when you add in the right inputs? It recalibrates. Quickly.

Each of these rituals helps you:

- Strengthen your gut lining
- Feed good bacteria
- Reduce gas and bloating
- Regulate your nervous system
- Poop more easily, consistently, and completely

It's not about being perfect. It's about being consistent enough for your body to remember what balance feels like.

. . .

Ayurvedic Spotlight

In Ayurveda, health is built on dinacharya daily habits that support your natural rhythms. Doing something small but intentional every day is more powerful than doing something intense once in a while.

When you pair warm food, mindful breathing, and supportive herbs with consistent routines, your body starts to trust you. It stops fighting. It opens up. It lets go emotionally and...literally.

Dr. Poop's Pro Tip

Start a Gut & Poop Diary. Track how you feel before and after meals. Note your energy, bloating, mood, and yes bowel movements. This isn't obsessive. It's data for you.

Ask yourself:

- Did that smoothie give me more energy?
- Did I poop more easily today?
- Was I less bloated after swapping pasta for lentils?
- Did 5 deep breaths calm my nerves before eating?

Open your mind to this whole body reconnection.

Final Word

Week 2 was about nourishment. You supported your gut bugs, added the good stuff in, and gave your insides a much-needed break from the noise.

But now it's time to go pro.

You've hydrated. You've moved. You've flushed.

Now, we're going to lock in the rhythm because consistent pooping isn't just about what you eat. It's about how you sit, how you breathe, when you go, and how safe your body feels.

Week 3 is your rhythm phase. You'll learn:

- The best position to poop (hint: it's not 90°)
- How to sync your bowels with your brain
- Why ghee might be your new bathroom buddy
- And how a little breathing can make a big difference

Your gut is ready. Your tools are primed.

Let's build a rhythm you can trust for life.

Onward to **Week 3: Poop Like a Pro**

3
WEEK 3: POOP LIKE A PRO

This week is your gut graduation. You're not just hoping for a good poop you're training your body to deliver it on cue. It's the difference between getting lucky... and getting consistent. You've cleared the funk, fed your microbiome, and now it's time to retrain your rhythm.

Think of this as Poop School for Adults where class starts in the bathroom, posture matters, and timing is everything.

This Week's Goal

Lock in regularity and master your body's natural poop cues.

Why It Works

Your body wants to poop regularly. But modern life throws that rhythm off. This week, we help your body remember how.

Let's break down the usual suspects behind poop delays:

- Dehydration: Not enough water = dry colon = poop bricks.
- Stress: Cortisol freezes digestion. When cortisol spikes, your digestion shuts down. Your body can't poop in fight-or-flight.
- Low Fiber Intake: Not enough roughage to form solid, smooth-moving poops.
- Toilet Posture: Sitting upright at a 90° angle kinks your rectum = blocked flow.
- Rushed Mornings: If you don't give your body time, it won't give you the signal.

Ayurvedic Spotlight

In Ayurveda, digestion is tied to the body's natural rhythms what you eat, when you eat, and how you eliminate. Morning elimination is considered a pillar of health, and any disturbance in that daily rhythm is a sign that your Agni (digestive fire) needs realignment.

This week, we embrace:

- Structured daily rituals to build bowel trust
- Posture and breath to help your body release safely
- Gentle internal lubricants like ghee to reduce strain

Dr. Poop's Pro Tip

If you've been winging your poop schedule, this is the week to schedule it. You train your dog to go out at the same time everyday, why not your bowels?

Let's poop with purpose. You're ready.

Up next: Rituals that train your brain and your bowels.

DR. POOP POSITIONS

Squat Position (The Poop Chute)

Goal: Straighten your poop chute and let gravity do the heavy lifting.

What It Is

This isn't yoga it's bathroom geometry. The squat position means elevating your feet (think: Squatty Potty, yoga blocks, a short stool) so your knees rise above your hips while you sit on the toilet. You're creating the angle your body was built to poop from.

Why It Works

In a seated position, your rectum is bent at a kinked angle, making you strain like you're lifting weights with your colon. But in a squat? That angle straightens out, allowing poop to slide out with less resistance.

This posture:

- Opens the anorectal canal
- Reduces straining and hemorrhoid risk
- Encourages a full release (no more "almost done" feelings)

Ayurvedic Spotlight

Ayurveda doesn't specifically mention Squatty Potties (they

didn't have TikTok in 5,000 BCE), but it does emphasize align-
ment, flow, and natural rhythms.

Squatting is:

- A natural posture that mirrors ancestral elimination
- A grounding pose that calms Vata energy (movement
  + nervous tension)
- Supportive of Apana Vayu the downward energy
  responsible for elimination

When your body feels aligned and grounded, it feels safe to
let go.

Dr. Poop's Pro Tip

Can't buy a Squatty Potty? Stack two hardcover books or flip your trash can upside down. The goal here is elevation, not aesthetics.

Lean Forward + Belly Hug (The Poop Factory)

Goal: Support natural elimination without strain.

What It Is

While sitting on the toilet, lean your torso slightly forward and gently press your hands into your lower abdomen right where your poop factory lives. Think of it like giving your gut a supportive nudge, not a shove.

Why It Works

This posture:

- Activates the abdominal wall without the need for force
- Encourages natural intra-abdominal pressure
- Mimics the fetal curl many of us instinctively move into during gut cramps (and for good reason)

It's a subtle hack to help your poop glide out more easily like turning on the "poop assist" feature your body already has.

Ayurvedic Spotlight

In Ayurveda, touch and awareness of the gut are believed to

awaken Agni (digestive fire) and stimulate Apana Vayu (the energy of downward elimination).

This practice:

- Grounds Vata energy
- Encourages energy to flow downward
- Calms the nervous system for safe release

In a world where we're always tensing and rushing, this ritual reminds your gut: You're supported. You're safe. You can let go.

Dr. Poop's Pro Tip

Pair this with deep breathing and a foot stool for the ultimate "no effort" release.

Knees-to-Chest Stretch (The Pre Poop Posture)

Goal: Activate your core and tell your pelvic floor it's go-time.

What It Is

Lay on your back, bring your knees toward your chest, and give yourself a gentle hug. Breathe into your belly as you hold for 30 seconds to 1 minute. This stretch can be done before your bathroom visit or anytime you feel stuck.

Why It Works

This pose:

- Activates your lower abdominal muscles, which help stimulate peristalsis
- Relaxes the pelvic floor, easing tension and supporting release
- Signals your gut-brain connection that it's time to let go

It's like a green light for your internal plumbing system.

Ayurvedic Spotlight

Ayurveda doesn't shy away from yoga as therapy. This pose aligns with Apanasana, the "wind-relieving pose" in yoga. It is often recommended to promote digestive flow.

Benefits:

- Balances Vata dosha
- Relieves gas and bloating
- Grounds the body and prepares it for elimination

Pair with belly breathing for added gut soothing effects.

Dr. Poop's Pro Tip

Do this first thing in the morning, before coffee or lemon water. Stack with Child's Pose if you're feeling especially blocked.

Child's Pose (Balasana)

Goal: Relieve gut tension and reset your nervous system to support a smooth release.

What It Is

Kneel on the floor, sit back on your heels, and fold your torso forward until your forehead rests on the ground. Arms can stretch forward or relax by your sides. Breathe deeply into your belly and lower back.

Use this pose any time you feel bloated, stuck, or "almost there" but not quite ready to go.

Why It Works

Child's Pose:

- Gently compresses the belly, massaging internal organs
- Stretches the lower back and spine, which often hold tension that blocks elimination
- Stimulates the vagus nerve, a key player in calming the gut-brain connection
- Tells your body: "You're safe. You can let go now."

This is your digestive timeout. A quiet, supported, and powerful space.

. . .

Ayurvedic Spotlight

In Ayurveda, balasana supports Apana Vayu the downward energy needed for elimination. The pose is often used to ground scattered energy, ease anxiety, and promote parasympathetic activation (rest + digest mode).

It's not just a yoga move. It's a bathroom warm-up.

Dr. Poop's Pro Tip:

Try this pose right before or after your knees to chest stretch. Bonus if you add calming breathwork to deepen the gut brain relaxation effect.

DAILY COMBO STACKS

The Stack Attack

Goal: Combine high-impact rituals for next-level morning success.

What It Is

Try this gut-boosting trifecta for smoother, more reliable mornings:

1. Take magnesium citrate or Triphala the night before
2. In the morning, use the squatting posture on the toilet
3. Layer in deep belly breathing for calm and coordination

Why It Works

This combo works on multiple levels:

- Magnesium or Triphala relaxes the colon overnight
- Squatting opens the rectal canal for easy passage
- Breathwork activates the parasympathetic nervous system, encouraging natural rhythm

Together, they form a synchronized system that clears the path, lowers resistance, and encourages the body to do what it already knows how to do.

. . .

Ayurvedic Spotlight

Ayurveda loves ritual stacks layering gentle habits that work in harmony.

This stack covers:

- Elimination (Apana Vayu)
- Digestion (Agni)
- Nervous system balance (Vata)

You're not just creating a routine you're building trust with your gut. Just the way Dr. Poop likes it!

Dr. Poop's Pro Tip

Do it at the same time every morning to train your gut like clockwork.

The Lemon Belly Breathing Combo

Goal: To train your body into a consistent, reliable poop schedule by stacking hydration, nervous system regulation, and timing all before breakfast.

What It Is

A daily stack: warm lemon water → deep belly breathing → consistent toilet time (same time every day).

Why It Works

Your body thrives on rhythm. When you do the same routine each morning, you condition your gut to expect action. Warm water stimulates the colon, breathwork activates the vagus nerve, and setting a consistent poop time strengthens your body's natural cues.

Ayurvedic Spotlight

Ayurveda emphasizes Dinacharya daily routines aligned with nature's rhythms. Pooping in the early morning (between 6–10 AM) is ideal, when Kapha energy is highest and elimination is easiest. Creating a predictable ritual in the morning reinforces balance across all doshas.

Dr. Poop's Pro Tip

Even if you don't feel the urge, sit and breathe. You're training your bowels the way you'd train a muscle. Keep the time sacred.

The Ghee Lubricator

Goal: To lubricate your digestive tract and jumpstart smooth, easy elimination first thing in the morning.

What It Is

Mix 1 teaspoon of ghee (clarified butter) into a cup of warm water and drink it first thing in the morning before breakfast.

Why It Works

Ghee lubricates the intestinal walls, supports bile flow, and nourishes your Agni (digestive fire), which helps your body process food more efficiently. Warm water hydrates and activates the gut lining, encouraging smoother, easier elimination. This combo gently preps your pipes for the day ahead like internal oiling.

Ayurvedic Spotlight

In Ayurveda, ghee is considered one of the most sacred digestive tonics.

It's known to:

- Strengthen Agni without aggravating Pitta
- Support the absorption of nutrients
- Calm the nervous system
- Heal and soothe the gut lining

This ritual is especially powerful for people with dry, hard stools or constipation linked to Vata imbalance.

Dr. Poop's Pro Tip

Use grass-fed or organic ghee if possible. If you're dairy-sensitive, start small ½ tsp and observe how your body responds.

The Prunes Psyllium Combo

Goal : To bulk up and soften your stool for easier, more regular poops

What It Is

Combine a few prunes (dried plums) with a teaspoon of psyllium husk mixed into water, juice, or a smoothie.

Why It Works

Prunes contain sorbitol, a natural sugar alcohol that pulls water into the intestines and acts like a gentle laxative. Psyllium is a soluble fiber that bulks up your stool and feeds your good gut bacteria. Together, they hydrate, soften, and move waste through your system like a well oiled machine.

Ayurvedic Spotlight

Ayurveda sees prunes as both nourishing and cleansing, perfect for balancing Vata and gently stimulating elimination. Psyllium (Isabgol) has long been used in India to improve bowel regularity without creating dependency or irritation.

Benefits of this combo:

- Eases incomplete elimination
- Reduces bloating by sweeping the colon
- Provides prebiotic fiber to support microbial diversity

Dr. Poop's Pro Tip

Soak your prunes in warm water for 15 minutes before eating if you want an even smoother effect. Don't forget to hydrate. Psyllium needs water to work!

DR. POOP'S WEEK 3 CHALLENGE

What It Is

Use the toilet at the same time every day this week, preferably in the morning. Choose 3 daily habits to stack (like lemon water, deep breathing, squatting posture). This is your practice zone. Train your gut like it's learning a dance choreography. Repetition builds rhythm.

Why It Works

Your gut loves a routine. Training your body to expect elimination at a certain time helps your brain activate those internal bathroom cues. Habit stacking creates a sensory signal (scent, sound, stretch, sip) that triggers gut motility like clockwork.

Ayurvedic Spotlight

Ayurveda champions Dinacharya daily rhythm that supports digestion, sleep, and overall health. Morning bowel movements are seen as a key part of detoxification, especially when you anchor them to gentle rituals like warm fluids, breathwork, and consistent timing.

This challenge supports:

- Strengthening your gastrocolic reflex
- Resetting your circadian digestive rhythm

- Building digestive trust and long-term regularity

Dr. Poop's Pro Tip

Before you eat anything in the morning, scrape your tongue. Scraping your tongue each morning is an ancient Ayurvedic ritual that removes overnight toxins, wakes up your digestion, and resets your gut for the day ahead.

Final Word

You've flushed, fed, and fine-tuned your gut. Now it's time to make it a lifestyle.

No more praying to the porcelain gods or Googling "how to poop faster" at 3 a.m.

Chapter 4 is your long-term maintenance plan. This is a toolbox of "Ayurvedic meets modern remedies" like olive oil shots, probiotic power ups, and bedtime lemon ginger rituals.

This is where your new habits harden into autopilot and your colon starts thanking you with clockwork-like poops. Ready to lock it in? Let's keep the flow going.

4
WEEK 4: MAINTAIN THE MOVEMENT

This week is your poop graduation. You've flushed the funk, fed the gut garden, and trained your body like a bowel boss. Now it's time to lock it in. The goal? Pooping with reliability, ease, and zero stress for life.

This Week's Goal

Maintain the momentum and solidify your new poop habits into a lifelong rhythm of smooth, stress-free digestion.

Why It Works

Temporary fixes are cute, but sustainable habits are where the real gut magic happens. When you consistently give your body the tools it needs hydration, movement, posture, and rhythm your digestive system adapts. You stop scrambling for last-minute solutions and start living in digestive peace.

Ayurvedic Spotlight

Ayurveda teaches samskara, or habit formation, as the key to long-term wellness. Once your gut is balanced, it thrives on daily rituals that honor your body's timing, energy, and needs. Consistency is the quiet healer.

This week supports:

- Solidifying your poop schedule
- Maintaining hydration and lubrication
- Reinforcing digestive trust and ease
- Preventing backslides into constipation chaos

Dr. Poop's Pro Tip

Don't chase "perfect poops." Chase peace of mind. When you treat your gut like a friend, not a fire to put out, you stay regular without overthinking it.

REMEDY 1: OLIVE OIL SHOT

What It Is

Take 1 teaspoon of cold-pressed extra virgin olive oil on an empty stomach ideally 20 to 30 minutes before your first meal.

You can follow it with warm water or add a splash of lemon for extra digestive power.

Why It Works

Olive oil acts like internal lube it softens stool, reduces friction during elimination, and signals your gallbladder to release bile (which helps break down fat and move things along). It's also rich in polyphenols that nourish your gut bacteria and reduce inflammation.

Ayurvedic Spotlight

In Ayurvedic tradition, internal oleation (snehana) is used to prep the body for cleansing. The oleation process helps loosen buildup, nourish tissues, and get things moving gently from the inside out. Ghee is commonly used, but olive oil is a modern-friendly option with similar benefits. Lubricating your GI tract first thing in the morning supports Agni (digestive fire) and regular elimination. Try it!

Dr. Poop's Pro Tip

If the oil alone grosses you out, chase it with lemon water or stir it into a warm drink. Imagine it's WD-40 for your colon, a smooth ride from start to flush.

REMEDY 2: PROBIOTIC POWER-UP

What It Is

Take a daily probiotic supplement with clinically studied strains like Lactobacillus reuteri, Bifidobacterium lactis, or Saccharomyces boulardii. My personal favorite is the brand Seed. If you prefer food-based options, reach for sauerkraut, kimchi, kefir, or miso.

Why It Works

Probiotics repopulate your gut with good bacteria that aid digestion, reduce inflammation, and improve stool regularity. They also crowd out harmful microbes that can slow your system down.

. . .

Ayurvedic Spotlight

Ayurveda recommends fermented dairy like lassi or fresh yogurt after meals to cool and balance digestion. Modern science confirms the benefits: more microbial diversity = more regular poops = happier gut.

Dr. Poop's Pro Tip

Make your probiotics part of a daily ritual, after breakfast or with your evening tea. And if you're more into food than pills, a spoonful of kimchi or kefir a day can do wonders.

Your gut isn't a solo act. It's a 100-trillion-member orchestra. Feed the musicians.

REMEDY 3: WARM LEMON GINGER WATER (PM)

What It Is

A cozy nighttime drink made with hot water, a few slices of fresh ginger, and the juice of half a lemon. Sip it slowly about an hour before bed.

Why It Works

This soothing combo hydrates your body overnight, supports bile flow, reduces bloating, and warms the digestive tract, helping your gut wind down and reset. Ginger is also a known stimulator of the vagus nerve, which plays a major role in triggering healthy bowel movements.

Ayurvedic Spotlight

Ginger and lemon are digestive powerhouses in Ayurveda. Ginger ignites Agni (your digestive fire), while lemon helps alkalize and cleanse. A warm, spiced beverage before bed is believed to support deep internal repair and reduce ama (toxins).

Dr. Poop's Pro Tip

Upgrade it with fennel seeds or chamomile for extra calm and gas relief. Think of this as your gut's bedtime story, steamy, citrusy, and soothing.

REMEDY 4: THE DAILY MOVEMENT PLEDGE

What It Is

Move your body for at least 10-30 minutes a day. Walk, stretch, do yoga, whatever feels doable. Bonus points if it happens after a meal or first thing in the morning.

Why It Works

Physical activity stimulates peristalsis (wave-like contractions that move food through your intestines) and triggers your gastrocolic reflex, the natural urge to poop after eating. Consistency builds rhythm.

Ayurvedic Spotlight

Ayurveda emphasizes vata-balancing movement like gentle walking or yoga to keep digestion flowing. Movement helps reduce stagnation and supports regular elimination, especially when paired with breath awareness.

· · ·

Dr. Poop's Pro Tip

Combine it with deep belly breathing and a brisk 5-minute post lunch walk for maximum effect. Think of it as your gut's favorite dance party.

REMEDY 5: RITUALIZED POOP TIME (YES, REALLY)

What It Is

Pick a consistent time each day, ideally within 30–60 minutes after a meal and commit to sitting on the toilet for 5–10 minutes. No scrolling, no distractions. Just you, your breath, and your body's natural cues.

Why It Works

Your brain and gut thrive on rhythm. By sitting at the same time daily, you train your body to expect elimination, kind of like potty Pavlov. This routine strengthens your natural gastrocolic reflex and builds digestive trust.

Ayurvedic Spotlight

According to Ayurveda, morning elimination (before 10 a.m.) is crucial for cleansing the body and aligning with circadian rhythms. Creating a sacred time and space for this process reinforces harmony between body and mind.

Dr. Poop's Pro Tip

Stack this time with supportive posture: elevate your feet (squat style), lean forward, and breathe deeply into your belly.

Add a gentle clockwise belly massage to really move things along. Make it sacred. Make it yours.

OPTIONAL DAILY HABIT STACKS

What It Is

Create repeatable, supportive routines by combining gut-friendly habits into morning and evening "stacks." These mini rituals become your gut groove, automatic, calming, and wildly effective.

Why It Works

Stacking habits triggers the brain to recognize patterns and stay consistent. It's the fastest way to turn relief into a lifestyle. Pairing habits with existing routines (like waking up or winding down) makes them stick.

Ayurvedic Spotlight

Ayurveda is rooted in Dinacharya, daily rituals that support optimal health. Morning routines ignite Agni and support elimination. Evening routines calm the nervous system, aiding rest and repair.

Dr. Poop's Pro Tip

Choose one stack to start:

- Morning Stack: Olive oil shot + warm water + squat posture + 5 minutes of quiet

- Evening Stack: Ginger tea + belly massage + probiotic + sleep
- Weekly Treat: Bone broth, foot massage, or an Epsom salt bath to calm your nervous system and pamper your gut

Mix, match, and repeat. This is how you make gut peace your new normal.

DR. POOP'S WEEK 4 CHALLENGE

What It Is

Pick 3 rituals from this week, olive oil shots, probiotics, poop-time rituals, you name it, and repeat them every day. Make it consistent. Make it yours. This isn't a cleanse. It's your new gut groove.

Why It Works

Repetition is where transformation lives. These habits aren't just short-term fixes, they're long-term investments in digestive ease. By locking in 3 that feel natural, you train your body to thrive without overthinking it.

Ayurvedic Spotlight

Ayurveda teaches that balance comes from rhythmic living. When your rituals align with your body's internal clock, your digestion, mood, and energy all improve. This week helps you anchor that rhythm.

. . .

Dr. Poop's Pro Tip

Keep it fun and visual: Track your rituals on a sticky note, phone app, or poop emoji chart. Seeing the streak builds momentum.

Bonus: reward yourself with something cozy (bath, foot rub, new squat stool name).

Final Word

By now, your gut isn't guessing, it's grooving. You've gone from stuck and sluggish to smooth and steady. But we're not ending with a flush... we're ending with freedom.

Let's close it out with a final pep talk, a few bonus rituals, and the truth bombs your colon's been waiting for.

5
BONUS CHAPTER: DR. POOP SMOOTHIES

When it comes to gut health, we often focus on what's on our plate, fiber rich veggies, probiotic-packed yogurts, healthy fats. But here's a secret weapon you might be overlooking: your cup. What you drink can be just as powerful (and sometimes even more effective) than what you eat.

Liquids are fast-absorbing, easier to digest, and incredibly soothing to a sensitive or sluggish gut. The right blends, whether whirred in a blender or steeped on your stovetop, can hydrate, calm, stimulate, and heal. They become your quiet allies. Your gentle reset buttons. Your "I need relief now" go-tos.

This bonus chapter is your cozy collection of gut-loving smoothies and tea rituals that are:

- Quick to make
- Full of natural, accessible ingredients
- Packed with gut-nourishing benefits
- Easy to prep ahead or grab on the go
- Kind to your taste buds *and* your colon

Whether you're blending something right before a walk, sipping something warm before bed, or reaching for a mid-day reset instead of your usual iced coffee, these recipes are here to keep you moving, in every sense of the word.

These aren't just drinks. They're functional tools for your digestion.

You'll find smoothies that:

- Lubricate and soften your stool (without cramping your style)
- Feed your gut microbes with fiber, prebiotics, and plant power
- Keep your blood sugar balanced so your mood (and bowels) don't crash

Most of the ingredients are pantry staples, ginger, mint, lemon, oats, chia, or banana. Others, like fennel, cardamom, or ghee, might become new favorites once you see how they help. And while the recipes are thoughtfully designed with your gut in mind, there's also plenty of room to customize, swap a fruit, add a spice, blend it thicker or thinner. There's no one right way to support your gut. These are simply starting points.

If you're busy (and let's face it, you probably are), these recipes are made to fit your life. No 40-minute prep times. No expensive powders. Just smart, simple blends you can toss together in under 5 minutes.

So let's sip your way to smoother movements. Use this chapter anytime you feel stuck, bloated, foggy, or just want to love your gut a little harder. You've done the work. You've flushed, fed, fine tuned, and maintained. Now it's time to enjoy the fruits (and herbs) of your labor.

Welcome to your new favorite habit: sipping for the sake of your gut.

Let's get blending and brewing.

SMOOTHIE #1: THE WARM FLUSH

What It Is

A warm smoothie for cold mornings or sluggish colons. Combines warming spices with fiber rich fruit to promote elimination.

Ingredients:

- 1/2 cooked apple (or pear)
- 1/2 banana
- 1/4 tsp cinnamon
- 1/4 tsp ground ginger
- 1 tbsp ground flaxseed
- 3/4 cup warm almond milk or oat milk

Blend until smooth and enjoy warm.

Why It Works

Warming spices activate digestion. Cooked fruit is easier on the gut than raw, and flaxseed adds gentle, effective fiber.

Ayurvedic Spotlight

This smoothie supports Agni (digestive fire) and reduces Vata, which is often elevated in constipation and cold digestion.

. . .

Dr. Poop's Pro Tip

Drink first thing in the morning to stimulate a bowel movement, especially helpful if your digestion is cold, slow, or stressed.

SMOOTHIE #2: GREEN MACHINE GO-TIME

What It Is

A refreshing fiber and mineral smoothie that tastes clean and helps clear sluggish systems.

Ingredients:

- 1 cup cucumber
- 1/2 avocado
- Handful of spinach
- Juice of 1/2 lemon
- 1/2 cup coconut water (or a dairy alternative milk)
- Pinch of sea salt

Blend and drink mid-morning or early afternoon.

Why It Works

Hydrating ingredients + magnesium + fiber = a powerful trifecta for moving the bowels and flushing excess bloat.

Ayurvedic Spotlight

This blend is Pitta-soothing and gently detoxifying without being harsh or drying.

Dr. Poop's Pro Tip

Add 1/4 tsp of psyllium husk if you're extra sluggish, but be sure to follow with a glass of water!

SMOOTHIE #3: CHOCOLATE CHIA BLISS

What It Is

A rich, dessert-y smoothie with chia seeds for fiber and magnesium, cacao for antioxidants, and dates for sweetness.

Ingredients:

- 1 cup almond milk
- 1 tbsp chia seeds
- 1 tbsp raw cacao powder
- 1–2 Medjool dates
- 1/2 frozen banana
- Optional: 1 scoop collagen or protein powder

Soak chia and dates for 10 mins, then blend everything.

Why It Works

Chia provides soluble fiber to bulk and soften stools. Cacao has magnesium to ease colon tension. Dates offer natural sweetness + prebiotic fiber.

Ayurvedic Spotlight

This is a grounding Kapha-friendly recipe that builds strength and supports gut motility without being overstimulating.

Dr. Poop's Pro Tip

Great for afternoon cravings or as a nourishing bedtime treat. Sip slowly with a spoon for mindful digestion.

SMOOTHIE #4: THE DIGESTIVE DREAM

What It Is

A simple, creamy blend that nourishes and supports slow or sensitive digestion.

Ingredients:

- 1/2 cup cooked oats
- 1/2 banana
- 1 tsp ghee or coconut oil
- Dash of cardamom
- 3/4 cup oat milk or almond milk

Blend and warm on stovetop or drink room temp.

Why It Works

Oats soothe the digestive lining. Ghee improves bile flow. This smoothie gently encourages elimination while stabilizing blood sugar. Try to find the brand MALK as they have no gum, no fillers, and no bad oils in their dairy alternative milks.

Ayurvedic Spotlight

Very Vata-calming, especially during dry seasons, travel, or stress.

Dr. Poop's Pro Tip

Use as a meal replacement when your gut feels raw or over-worked. It's pure comfort.

SMOOTHIE #5: THE PINEAPPLE GINGER GLOW-UP

What It Is

A zesty, enzyme-rich smoothie that wakes up your digestion and reduces post-meal bloat.

Ingredients:

- 1/2 cup pineapple (fresh/frozen)
- 1/2 banana
- Small slice of fresh ginger
- Juice of 1/2 lime
- 1 tbsp ground flaxseed
- Water or coconut water to blend

Why It Works

Pineapple's bromelain supports protein digestion. Ginger promotes GI movement. Flax supports stool bulk and ease.

Ayurvedic Spotlight

This smoothie activates digestion and clears excess Kapha. Great after heavier meals.

Dr. Poop's Pro Tip

Use this mid-morning to re-energize your system and help regulate afternoon elimination.

SMOOTHIE #6: THE CREAM PIE

What It Is

A creamy, dessert-like smoothie packed with healthy fats and magnesium to help you go before bed.

Ingredients:

- 1 ripe banana
- 1 tbsp tahini
- 1/2 tsp cinnamon
- 1/2 tsp vanilla extract
- 1 cup almond milk
- Optional: 1–2 soaked dates

Why It Works

Tahini (sesame seeds) is rich in minerals. Bananas are soothing and naturally sweet. Helps move things along overnight.

Ayurvedic Spotlight

Great for dry, slow-moving bowels and supportive of hormone balance.

Dr. Poop's Pro Tip

Add a pinch of sea salt to boost absorption and flavor. This one tastes like dessert and works like medicine.

Final Word

Let's dive into the world of magical teas now!

6

BONUS CHAPTER: DR. POOP TEAS

Sipping is underrated. Teas are fast-acting, gut-soothing little potions that deliver warmth, hydration, and powerful plant magic straight to your digestive system. They slip past sluggish digestion and go to work fast. They calm nerves, ease cramps, reduce bloat, and nurture your body into its natural rhythm.

This is your steeped survival kit. Your backup plan when dinner didn't sit right. Your nightly hug-in-a-mug. Whether you're dealing with bloating, constipation, or just want to wind down and poop like a pro, these tea rituals are here for you.

These daily digestive rituals:

- Calm your vagus nerve and activate your "rest and digest" mode
- Reduce gas, bloating, and belly pressure
- Stimulate bile and enzyme flow for smoother, easier digestion
- Turn into comforting habits you actually look forward to

. . .

So put the kettle on. Let's sip our way to gut greatness.

TEA #1: LET IT FLOW LAVENDER

What It Is

A calming tea to wind down your nervous system and support overnight digestion.

Ingredients:

- 1 chamomile tea bag
- 1/2 tsp dried lavender
- Optional: lemon slice or honey

Why It Works

Chamomile reduces inflammation and cramps. Lavender calms your vagus nerve and promotes restful poops.

Ayurvedic Spotlight

Deeply Vata-soothing and ideal for stress-induced sluggishness.

Dr. Poop's Pro Tip

Drink this while doing a gentle belly massage before bed. Add soft music or a candle to complete the ritual.

TEA #2: GINGER MINT WAKE-UP

What It Is

A bright, invigorating tea to start your digestive fire and reduce sluggishness or morning bloat.

Ingredients:

- 1-inch fresh ginger (sliced or grated)
- 4–5 fresh mint leaves (or 1 mint tea bag)
- Juice of 1/4 lemon
- Optional: dash of cayenne or honey

Steep in hot water for 5–7 minutes. Strain and sip slowly.

Why It Works

Ginger boosts circulation and motility. Mint soothes the GI tract. Lemon kickstarts bile production and detoxification.

Ayurvedic Spotlight

A digestion-stimulating blend that balances Kapha and awakens Agni (digestive fire).

Dr. Poop's Pro Tip

Drink 15–30 minutes before breakfast to support easier, more complete elimination later in the morning.

TEA #3: THE BLOAT BUSTER

What It Is

A gently aromatic tea that targets bloating, gas, and that "why-do-I-feel-so-massive" post-lunch sensation.

Ingredients:

- 1 tsp fennel seeds
- 2 crushed cardamom pods
- Optional: 1/4 tsp coriander seeds or fresh orange peel

Simmer in 1.5 cups of water for 8–10 minutes. Strain and enjoy warm.

Why It Works

Fennel relaxes the intestines and eases gas. Cardamom supports healthy enzyme production and eases cramping. Together, they reset your gut without harshness.

Ayurvedic Spotlight

A Tridoshic tea, balanced enough for all doshas. Especially helpful after heavy or rushed meals.

Dr. Poop's Pro Tip

Keep a small jar of the seed blend in your pantry and steep a fresh batch anytime bloating hits.

Final Word

Sadly, it's that time to close our beautiful poop journey together...turn the page.

CLOSING REFLECTION: WHY SIPPING MATTERS

S ips are sacred. They're not just fuel, they're signals. Every time you pause to blend a smoothie or steep a tea, you're telling your nervous system, "Hey, we're safe. You can digest now."

In a world of chug-and-go energy drinks and meal replacements, these small rituals, these warm, nourishing sips, help soften inner chaos, reduce inflammation, and remind your gut of its rhythm.

So don't just sip for symptom relief.

Sip because you're worth slowing down for.

Sip because your gut deserves luxury.

Sip because healing is an inside job.

Let your drinks be medicine.

Let your moments be sacred.

And never forget, your gut's greatest power comes not from force, but from flow.

THE FINAL FLUSH

DECLARATION
Let's be clear: what you just did wasn't small.

You didn't just try a few health tips. You showed up for yourself, every single day for 30 days. You learned how to nourish, listen to, and work with your body instead of fighting it. You took back control from the chaos, confusion, and constipation that ruled your mornings (and sometimes your whole week).

You didn't need another quick fix, a shady supplement, or a six-week bootcamp that treats your body like a machine. You needed rhythm. You needed rituals. And you delivered. With oils, teas, squats, and walks. You delivered.

You are now, officially, a Poop Pro.

Not because you hit perfection, but because you learned to partner with your gut instead of punishing it. Most people never learn this!

· · ·

REMINDER

Let's remember what's actually changed here.

Your gut isn't just a digestive tube, it's your body's second brain. It talks to your mood, your immunity, your energy, your hormones, your skin, and your stress. It tells you, every single day, how you're actually doing, no filter, no sugarcoat.

And now? You actually know how to listen.

You've swapped punishment for patience. You've replaced guesswork with grounded habits. You've learned that a warm mug of ginger tea can sometimes do more than an expensive powder with 12 syllables. You've stopped looking for magic pills and started building consistent routines.

The daily rituals you practiced, whether it was olive oil in the morning, movement after lunch, or belly breathing before bed weren't just gut helpers. They were nervous system whispers. They were acts of devotion. They were reminders that self care doesn't have to be sexy to be sacred.

SHIFT

What you've done isn't temporary. This wasn't a diet. This was a reset, and that means your entire relationship with your gut has shifted. Permanently.

Sure, you'll have off days. Travel will throw you off. Work will get stressful. You'll eat something weird at 11 p.m. and question your life choices. But now, you have tools. You have rituals to come home to. You don't spiral anymore you re-center.

You now know that rhythm goes hand and hand with willpower.

That hydration beats deprivation.

That poop doesn't have to be a mystery, it can be a mirror.

You stopped chasing fast fixes and started building slow magic. And that's what makes it sustainable.

FORWARD VISION

This is not the end. This is your gut's new beginning.

From here, you get to decide: What rituals will you keep? What foods make you feel truly good? What daily habits help you stay in flow physically, emotionally, spiritually?

You don't have to do everything perfectly. You don't need to remember every tip in this book. But you do need to remember how it felt when your gut was finally on your side. Keep chasing that feeling.

Keep stacking rituals. Keep flushing shame. Keep experimenting. Keep laughing when your squat stool falls over or your partner catches you belly massaging in the mirror. Keep walking after dinner. Keep sipping warm tea instead of scrolling. Keep trusting that your body wants to feel better, and now knows how.

And most of all, keep coming back to yourself. Because the biggest gift of this 30-day reset isn't a perfect poop, it's the quiet, steady confidence that you can feel better...every single day.

You didn't just poop better.

You lived better.

And you always can.

With deepest respect (and a wink),

- Dr. Poop A.K.A. "Constipation's Worst Nightmare"

P.S. - bring this book with you wherever you go so you can always poop like a pro!

. . .

P.P.S. - if this book helped you improve just one thing in your life, please pay it forward and share with a friend. You could change their life, one poop at a time.

BIBLIOGRAPHY

Axe, Josh. *Eat Dirt: Why Leaky Gut May Be the Root Cause of Your Health Problems and 5 Surprising Steps to Cure It*. Harper Wave, 2016.

Bulsiewicz, Will. *Fiber Fueled: The Plant-Based Gut Health Program for Losing Weight, Restoring Your Health, and Optimizing Your Microbiome*. Avery, 2020.

Chutkan, Robynne. *The Microbiome Solution: A Radical New Way to Heal Your Body from the Inside Out*. Avery, 2015.

DeLaney, Megan. "What You Should Know About Triphala." *Cleveland Clinic Health Essentials*, 2022. https://health.clevelandclinic.org/triphala

Gershon, Michael. *The Second Brain: A Groundbreaking New Understanding of Nervous Disorders of the Stomach and Intestine*. Harper Perennial, 1999.

Gottfried, Sara. *The Hormone Cure*. Scribner, 2013.

Hari, Johann. *Lost Connections: Uncovering the Real Causes of Depression – and the Unexpected Solutions*. Bloomsbury, 2018.

Kharrazian, Datis. *Why Isn't My Brain Working?*. Elephant Press, 2013.

Mayo Clinic Staff. "Constipation." *Mayo Clinic*, 2021. https://www.mayoclinic.org/diseases-conditions/constipation

Mayo Clinic Staff. "Magnesium Supplements." *Mayo Clinic*, 2022. https://www.mayoclinic.org/drugs-supplements-magnesium

National Institute of Diabetes and Digestive and Kidney Diseases. "Symptoms & Causes of Constipation." *NIDDK*, 2020. https://www.niddk.nih.gov/health-information/digestive-diseases/constipation

Singh, Ram Harsh. *Foundations of Ayurveda: Ancient Insights for Modern Times*. Chaukhambha Surbharti Prakashan, 2009.

Spector, Tim. *The Diet Myth: The Real Science Behind What We Eat*. Orion Publishing, 2015.

University of Maryland Medical Center. "Psyllium." *UMMC Complementary and Alternative Medicine Guide*. https://www.umm.edu/health/medical/altmed/herb/psyllium

Wells, Georgia Ede. "How to Calm the Anxious Gut." *Psychology Today*, 2022. https://www.psychologytoday.com/us/blog/diagnosis-diet/202202/how-calm-the-anxious-gut